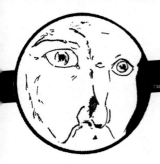

MW01104230

The Psychology of Retirement:

How to Cope
Successfully with a
Major Life Transition

by The Everyday Psychologist

Premier Edition: Includes the
self-scoring *Retirement Stress Inventory*

BPRI Press

Business Psychology Research Institute
The Everyday Psychology Series: Volume 2
836 East Rand Road, PMB #274
Arlington Heights, IL 60004
phone 847/255-5481 ■ fax 847/255-3480
WWW.BPRI.COM ■ BPRI2000@AOL.COM

Library of Congress
Catalog Card Number: 99-091209

ISBN: 0-9668417-2-7

Book design: Kim Allen-Hohman
Illustration: Alexander D. Jones

Printed in the United States of America

BPRI PRESS

Contents

.

Preface

.
.
.

This book series is titled *The Everyday Psychology Series*. Anonymous psychologists who specialize in the topics of concern will write each edition in this series. Therefore it should be no surprise to anyone that the pseudonym that was adopted for this book series is The Everyday Psychologist.

BPRI Press wants the focus of this series to be on cutting-edge psychological theories, interventions, and insights, and not on the authors! However, each book that is anonymously authored for BPRI Press will include a reference section that will list many of the best known studies in the field of inquiry that the self-help book addresses. Readers can go to these original sources if they are interested in learning more about the teachings of a particular researcher or psychologist. There are three major goals for *The Everyday Psychology Series*:

- *To cover psychological topics that can help readers to cope better with the pressures of the new millennium.*

- *To base each book on scientific findings as much as possible, so that readers will be better informed about the topic of concern.*

- *Finally, to publish brief, user-friendly books so that readers can quickly learn new skills and strategies that can help them cope better with their lives.*

■ *In short, BPRI Press does not want to publish books that are perceived to be excessively academic in nature.*

We have one word of caution. By attempting to simplify and summarize complicated research studies and interpretations, the authors will surely leave out some important details that readers might really want to study. Hopefully readers will use the list of resources in the reference section for this purpose. Still, any self-help material presented in *The Everyday Psychology Series* is for informational purposes only, and should not be used for making any form of clinical or treatment decisions. Moreover, it is this editorial board's opinion that physicians or mental health professionals should always be consulted whenever a person is experiencing a serious problem in living. This includes physical, mental, emotional, and even spiritual problems.

With this second volume of *The Everyday Psychology Series*, it is important to point out that all retirees will experience retirement differently. This self-help book simply lists some research-based "red flags" that usually need to be addressed before it is possible to achieve a high-level positive retirement. Examples of red flags include poor health status before retirement, retiring earlier than planned, lacking knowledge about the retirement process, and experiencing a general dissatisfaction with life, to name a few. Readers will also learn how to view retirement as a normal life transition rather than a stressful life event. Finally, *The Psychology of Retirement* includes a listing of Web sites that cater to the specific needs of retirees.

Editorial Board
BPRI Press
September 22, 1999

The Psychology of Retirement:

How to Cope Successfully with a Major Life Transition

■
Introduction
■

The Psychology of Retirement addresses retirement stress and what to do about it. This self-help book is relevant to both retirees and not-yet-retirees, along with their families and significant others. This publication:

■ *Explains some major life adjustment issues that retirees routinely face*

■ *Discusses key emotional reactions to retirement*

■ *Provides information that, if applied, can make the retirement process smooth and enjoyable for retirees and their families*

A word of caution is required. *The Psychology of Retirement* should be viewed as supplemental information only. It is not a panacea and should not be used as a replacement for any form of medical and/or psychological treatment that retirees and their families might require. Also, this publication is relevant to retirees in general; it should not be taken as a prescription for any particular person. Now, let's begin! We will first explore the two basic views that people have about retirement.

■
Retirement as a Stressful Life Event
■

Retirement can be seen as a stressful life event. Why
stressful? Because you're losing something very important
in your life: your job! Nearly all employees make a major
investment of their time and egos when it comes to their jobs
and careers. This loss may trigger physical and emotional
stress. Consider the following statements, which definitely
support the notion that retirement is a stressful life experience:

"Retirement is the ugliest word in the language."

ERNEST HEMINGWAY, AMERICAN AUTHOR

*"Americans hardly ever retire from business: they are
either carried out feet first or they jump from the
window."*

PROFESSOR A. L. GOODHART, AMERICAN LAWYER

*"Have you ever been out for a late autumn walk in the
closing part of the afternoon, and suddenly looked up to
realize that the leaves have practically all gone? And
the sun has set and the day gone before you knew it—
and with that a cold wind blows across the landscape?
That's retirement."*

STEPHEN LEACOCK, CANADIAN HUMORIST AND ECONOMIST

*"Few men (or women) have been able to make a
graceful exit at the appropriate time."*

MALCOLM MUGGERIDGE, BRITISH JOURNALIST

Many other losses are associated with retirement. For
instance, economic loss: you don't have the steady paycheck

to count on each week. However, this is less of an issue for those employees who have financially planned for a stable retirement.

Next, you may feel a loss of status. This is especially true for high-level executives who have been at the top of the mountain for a long time. They have contributed to their company for many, many years, building up a lot of well-earned status. If that sounds like you, accept the fact that it's natural—it's OK—to feel a sense of loss over giving up one's executive status.

Most important to retirees is activity loss. For a very long time, forty hours—or more—of your life each week have been tied to one basic activity: your job, your career! For executives, that included running a company, making key decisions, interacting with employees and shareholders, and basically seeing the ups and downs, the highs and lows of those efforts. The psychological impact of losing 40 hours or more of activity each week should not be minimized!

Finally, you can face identity loss. Many people associate who they are with their career. If you are an executive, you identify with the fact that you are in charge, you run the company, and you are constantly looked up to by your staff. Therefore, oftentimes when you retire, a dominant part of your identity—your image of who you are—can be greatly affected.

Retirement is just one of many stressful life changes that retirees might encounter. People who are retiring may have other changes going on in their lives at the same time. Such people are at a much higher risk for stress-related illness, injury, or some other type of loss. However, of all such changes that may be taking place, retirement is one of the most challenging of the stressful life events.

Assessing Your Retirement Stress Level

You will find an informal self-assessment stress questionnaire in Appendix A. Called the *"Retirement Stress Inventory,"* it consists of 20 questions. Shortly, I'll ask you to complete and score that questionnaire. You will be able to add up your answers and determine your predisposition for a stress-related illness or injury.

For example, if you score extremely low on the inventory, the odds are lower that you will have any significant stress-related health problems related to retirement. However, if you score extremely high, you have a much higher chance of developing a stress-related illness or injury during retirement. As a general rule of thumb, If you score in the higher risk ranges (e.g., 21 or higher), then it's very important that you work hard to manage your stress and to minimize any more stressful life changes. Also, if you score in the higher risk ranges, it might be in your best interest to consult a physician and/or clinical counselor.

What types of illnesses have been associated with extremely high scores on this type of stress inventory? Some of the more serious examples are heart disease and hypertension, depression and chronic fatigue, gastrointestinal disorders, muscular aches and pains, low resistance to infection, proneness to accidents, sexual dysfunction, and a flare-up of preexisting medical disorders such as hypertension, alcoholism, and diabetes. Research has even linked chronic and excessive levels of stress to the onset of cancer. Finally, a few severely distressed people who can't cope with their stressful life events might even consider suicide!

Obviously, becoming aware of all the major life changes currently affecting your health is vitally important. So please take the time now to complete the self-assessment questionnaire located in Appendix A. Remember to compute your score so that you can become more aware of your risk for stress-related problems during your pre-retirement and retirement years. (Note: Because the questionnaire in Appendix A provides a very informal assessment of retirement stress, readers who want a more precise measure of stress are encouraged to take a scientifically validated stress assessment from a licensed psychologist or counselor.)

Managing Your Retirement Stress Level

Thank you for completing the questionnaire and computing your score. As stated above, higher scores are usually related to an increased risk for stress-related illness.

What should you do now? If you obtained an exceptionally high stress score, the main thing to keep in mind is that you might be at a high risk for some type of stress-related illness. Therefore, please consult a physician or counselor. Are you in shape to deal with increased stress? Are you overweight? Do you have hypertension? Are you abusing alcohol or drugs? These questions and others need to be answered. Of course, since this is an informal stress assessment, even people who score lower on the questionnaire might benefit from getting a comprehensive medical checkup. In addition, some people who score in the higher risk ranges might be perfectly healthy.

Practicing some type of stress management and wellness program is also important. Overly stressed retirees must take the time each day to improve their health and coping skills. Proper weight control and nutrition are crucial for retirees, too. Check with your physician to make sure you are getting the proper vitamin intake and nutrition. A high score on the stress questionnaire means that the stress in your life, whether you acknowledge it or not, could be robbing your body of needed nutrients. You then become, over time, even more susceptible to stress-related illness.

Light exercise is also important. Keep your body fit and stay in shape. If physically possible, take healthy walks, jog short distances, and even swim. Engage in light calisthenics, or rhythmic exercise. Keep your body healthy and strong so that it can buffer the effects of stress. (Caution: Obtain a physical examination from a qualified health professional before engaging in any type of exercise, fitness, or wellness program.)

Retirees must also reduce or eliminate smoking, drinking, and other forms of substance abuse. No one can say that you are definitely at risk for alcoholism or chemical dependency during retirement. However, some people dealing with retirement stress are more likely to mistakenly use alcohol and other mood-altering drugs as a way to cope and relax. Instead, you can use more healthful, less dangerous forms of relaxation (e.g., exercising, meditating, prayer). For an example, see Appendix B for a progressive relaxation script for retirees who experience a lot of physical tension. And please, consult a clinical counselor or self-help counseling program if you are at risk for any type of substance abuse!

On a side note, many retirees start to shift the blame for all of their problems to the retirement process itself. However, if you had problems in the previous, career, phase of your life, you are also at risk to have problems in retirement! Saying that those problems were caused by retirement is unfair. The truth is that any preexisting problems in living run the risk of being aggravated by retirement. Retirees still have the responsibility to get at the root causes of all their problems and start correcting them.

■

Retirement as a Normal Life Transition

■

A second, more positive way to view the retirement process is that retirement is a normal life transition. In other words, don't label retirement as a crisis situation; instead, view it as an accepted social role. You are merely moving from one phase of life to another. In the old phase, many of your activities revolve around your job and the workplace. In the new phase of life as a retiree, you have increased leisure time.

Your primary challenge during retirement is to find substitute activities in your daily routine that are very interesting and important to you and that will give your life meaning and purpose. These substitute activities should not be trivial, and they may not be easy to discover. You might go through much trial and error. And that's not unusual.

Emotional adjustment to retirement typically goes through four stages: (1) denial, (2) depression, (3) anger, and (4) acceptance. Figure 1 visually displays these four distinct phases of the retirement process. You will more than likely go through these four phases as a retiree, and your family members and others closely related to you are likely to go through them, too. Retirees normally go through all four phases.

Phase I: Denial. When you start working toward or begin living in retirement, you'll likely want very much to deny that retirement will create great changes physically, emotionally, and socially. The denial process deserves a close look. In this stage, you begin to isolate yourself from others, including family, friends, and coworkers. The isolation doesn't necessarily have to be social; it might be emotional, too. You are feeling a struggle inside yourself, and such feelings are usually a required step when adjusting to the retirement process.

Another form of denial is to internalize feelings such as anger, resentment, and fear, to name a few. You are making a very normal life transition; yet at some level, whether it's conscious or unconscious, you do not totally trust everyone around you. Keep in mind, you feel some status loss, and you are moving to a new phase of life where you might not be the expert. It's natural to internalize your feelings at this point. Some people even minimize their role loss, saying, "Hey, this retirement thing is easy. I'll have no problems, and it should be very easy to cope." That is probably true for some people. However, all retirees will go through, in some degree, each emotional stage of the retirement process.

Retirees in denial do not yet accept that retirement marks the end of a major life commitment: their jobs! Part of the denial process is to minimize both the size and the complexity of your decisions during the retirement phase of life. However, you are looking for ways to live the rest of your life. New activities will be needed to help bring meaning to your life. This takes much time, thought, and planning.

Another form of denial is unrealistic expectations or catastrophic thinking. You may feel retirement should be more enjoyable than it really is, and you feel let down when those unrealistic expectations are not fulfilled. Catastrophic thoughts include the following: "Retirement is terrible. My life isn't meaningful. I will never have a meaningful life again." Nonsense! You have to brainstorm and become creative in order to determine those activities that will give your life new meaning. Embrace this responsibility fully and get on with this new phase of your life.

Figure 1

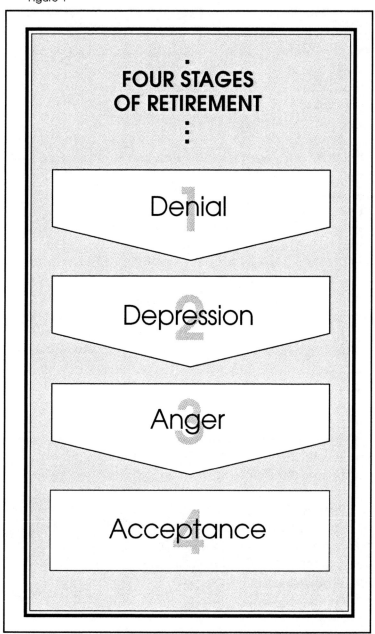

FOUR STAGES
OF RETIREMENT

Denial 1

Depression 2

Anger 3

Acceptance 4

Phase II: Depression. After denial, some form of depression typically sets in. In the denial phase of retirement, you were not dealing with all of the challenges of retirement because you were minimizing the transition. However, in the depression phase, you start allowing yourself to experience those feelings of being overwhelmed. This is a natural occurrence.

Since many people do not really know what depression is, let's review some of its features for retirees. First, you begin to feel sad and downhearted over the loss of your job and career. You feel, "Hey, this is a very drastic and serious change for me, and I'm not sure I can handle it." You know you are moving away from a life activity that has been very important for a long time: your job, your career. You might regretfully acknowledge that you did not fully accomplish everything you wanted to do in your career. That is natural. No one is perfect, and no one can accomplish everything. You just have not yet learned to accept this reality!

You might begin to feel overwhelmed with all the issues that you must eventually cope with during retirement. You may engage in increased substance abuse (e.g., alcohol, drugs, and food) during this phase to soothe some of the emotional anguish you are feeling. Keep in mind that you might not be aware that you have a slight depression; so examine your activity level. Also seek feedback from family and friends. Are you withdrawing? Are you doing less?

You might even be experiencing a biochemical stress reaction. By that I mean you are probably more fatigued than normal. You might not have a lot of energy. Your entire body might feel drained from the stress. Loss of social and sexual interest can occur—and not because your mate is undesirable or you are undesirable. It is because you are experiencing the retirement stress syndrome (e.g., you are preoccupied with and overly worried about your retirement).

Parenthetically, one of the major signs that you are experiencing either a slight or more serious depression is that you have a feeling of what we call an "existential crisis." That is, your retirement makes you aware that you are reaching a later stage of the life cycle. For many, this is a truly disturbing reality! They do not feel their life has any meaning or purpose. These feelings of despair will need to be acknowledged, understood, and eventually worked through.

As indicated above, you may continue to withdraw from people, activities, and associations. In fact, you will probably decrease your overall level of activity in general. This is quite understandable. You are not yet emotionally prepared to start building the retirement phase of your life.

Phase III: Anger. Ironically, one way out of depression is to begin to recognize and express your pent-up feelings of anger. When working with depressed clients, therapists usually view it as progress whenever a depressed person starts to express anger. This is a hopeful sign that the depression has a better chance of lifting.

How can you know if you are in the anger phase of the retirement process? First, you might start blaming others for your predicament (e.g., your spouse, your children, your in-laws, and other significant others). Everyone else is to blame for somehow coercing you into retirement. You will probably blame your employer, too. Your company did not fully support you in this transition. They let you go too soon. They did not ask you to stay on as long as you would have liked. And you don't leave out your boss. You might decide your boss is the source of all the trying emotional times that you are going through right now.

Another way of being angry is subtler. Because you feel frustrated yourself, you start demanding quicker adjustments to your retirement from your family members. Since focusing on your own needs during retirement is so uncomfortable, you focus on their needs and spend your energy trying to manage their emotional adjustment to retirement stress. Stop! Detach yourself! Let all your family members and loved ones work on their own emotional adjustment at their own pace. If everyone is having serious problems adjusting to your retirement, then a meeting with a professional counselor should probably be scheduled.

Next, you might resist certain family activities, such as your spouse working when you are retired. Duties might be reassigned in the home. For example, a recently retired spouse might take on some of a nonworking spouse's chores at home, causing the nonworking spouse to feel threatened. Or the retired spouse will be asked to take on some chores of a still-working spouse, which can make for a very resentful retiree. Other family members might also feel threatened if the retiree takes over some of their household duties and responsibilities. In brief, the retiree's plans are tampering with the equilibrium of the entire family system.

The anger phase also produces the tendency to "regress" and "act out" by demanding extra sympathy. Do retirees directly ask for sympathy? No, of course not, but their moods and behaviors seem to be calls for some statements of sympathy, either from friends, work colleagues, or family members. Also, recent retirees or those facing that change might do things they never did before, such as staying out late repeatedly or ignoring the family. Some might even make the family their "new job." They might try to attempt to manage the family members the same way they managed their company. Do not do it!

What's really happening is that you are beginning to vent your anger, which will allow you to take steps emotionally toward growth and understanding of the retirement process. Feeling angry is therefore a good sign! A healthy sign!

Make sure you do not get stuck in the anger stage. The deep underlying feelings that retirees have to acknowledge is that they are somewhat scared and insecure about their new role. And there is nothing wrong with those feelings. Accept them! Embrace them! Work through them! And then move on! Accept the challenge of retirement and move forward.

Phase IV: Acceptance. Work through that anger, and you are ready to move into the final phase: full acceptance of and adjustment to retirement. Now you must develop actual plans for day-to-day retirement activities.

Many retirees meticulously planned much of their work life, and now they must plan the retirement phase of their life in the same careful, thorough manner. This means increasing day-to-day activities to fill "the retirement vacuum." If you accept the challenge of retirement in the same way you accepted the challenge of thousands of exciting work projects, this can be a real adventure.

Most important, do not force family adjustment. The entire family is adjusting to your retirement, and that process can take many months. Often during the acceptance and adjustment phase, retirees and their spouses might need to seek outside professional help, such as a crisis counselor or retirement coach. And retirees should certainly seek outside help if they feel things are not going the way they would like them to go. It may be a humbling experience, but retirees who need help must reach out for it—for their own well being and for the well being of their loved ones.

What a shame when retirees live the next 20, 30, maybe 40 or more years not fully satisfied with this, the retirement, phase of their lives! If you can adjust to all four phases of retirement—denial, depression, anger, and acceptance—then you have worked toward a truly satisfying, high-level retirement. Let us now turn our attention to major warning signs that suggest difficulties in coping with retirement stress.

■

Retirement Stress Warning Signs

■

The first warning sign of poor adjustment to retirement is length of adjustment. Working through the stages of denial, depression, anger, and acceptance—and thus full adjustment to retirement—usually takes a number of months, six to nine on average. If the process takes an excessively long time—if, for example, you are taking over a year to develop and implement your retirement plan—then touch base with a retirement counselor who can help you get on track.

Another warning sign of a poor adjustment to retirement is difficulty keeping busy with meaningful activities. The new activities in your life must be meaningful and planned. They must be things you want to do not something other people have forced down your throat. In fact, people need a schedule of day-to-day activities more in the retirement phase of their lives than in the work phase. Why? Because the retirement phase by itself is less structured, so more structure needs to be developed.

A third major warning sign of poor adjustment is dissatisfaction with retirement in general, an overall feeling of dissatisfaction and discontent with being out of the workforce. You worry excessively about not working; you miss many of your work colleagues and job duties; you fantasize a lot about your old job. If such feelings, wishes, and desires are chronic and distracting, then you are adjusting poorly to retirement.

Another warning sign is intense family tension over retirement. You adopt the feeling as a retiree of "it's me against them." Not only do you isolate yourself from your family but you become defensive, too. You stop working toward full acceptance, on an emotional level, of your retirement.

The final major sign of poor adjustment is that health complications—mental, emotional, or physical—begin to occur. If you are having increased health problems of any sort, a medical evaluation is definitely recommended. You probably cannot work out these health issues on your own. Next, we'll review some of the predictors of a healthy adjustment to retirement.

■

Predictors of Adjustment

■

Retirement stress is caused not only by the loss of a job but by a number of related factors. These factors are known as the predictors of adjustment.

Red Flags. Some factors are potential "red flags" that something can go wrong with your retirement process. Let us discuss some of these red flags.

Health status. Health status is the first, most important factor that impacts the quality of your retirement. Poor health before retirement often leads to poor health during retirement. *Researchers show that most people who have serious health complications during retirement had them before retirement, too. So, if you have been healthy before retirement, chances are you will enjoy a healthier lifestyle during retirement.*

Financial status. *Retirement is more difficult, and more stressful, if the personal and family budget is tight. Everybody, wealthy and not so wealthy alike, needs the security of careful financial planning during retirement. The sense of security it brings creates a higher-quality retirement.*

Early retirement. *Another potential red flag is a retirement that was earlier than planned. If you planned the date of your retirement and are retiring when you wanted to retire, then chances are you will have fewer complaints and complications than people do who retired because the company either forced— or highly encouraged—them to retire earlier than they wanted.*

Desirability of retirement. *People who do not really want to retire become more stressed than do people who truly desire retirement. So, if deep down you know you do not want to retire, even if you act like you want it you will probably be more distressed than people who actually do want to retire.*

Family stability and support. *Retirees living in stable, supportive families have an easier time adjusting than do retirees living in unsupportive or even antagonistic families. If any source of tension is affecting your family, seek help to correct it. Your retirement process will become more enjoyable.*

Marital status. *Research has shown that retirees who are divorced, separated, or widowed have a* *harder time with retirement, compared with retirees still living with their spouses. Retirees with companions have a much easier time adjusting. If you are divorced, separated, or widowed, you absolutely need to seek strong, supportive friendships and community involvement to ease your retirement transition.*

Social support network. *Isolated retirees have a more difficult time adjusting than retirees who are fully involved with family and community networks do. If you do not have a strong social support group, make the effort to develop one.*

General dissatisfaction with life. *People who are dissatisfied with life before retirement will most likely continue to have morale problems during retirement. Retirement isn't the culprit here; these disillusioned retirees need a positive change in attitude, or they will be as dissatisfied in retirement as they were before.*

Incomplete knowledge about retirement. *Uninformed retirees have the most difficulties. Hopefully, you will become better able to cope with retirement after reading The Psychology of Retirement. At bookstores and libraries, you can find other books to help you understand what to expect and how to resolve specific problems you may encounter. Take the time to read these, and you will be the better retiree for that. Also local community colleges and other groups in your area will likely offer programs to help with retirement planning.*

Heavy involvement with work. *Work can be like an addiction to many. Most executives and other retirees who were deeply, deeply involved with their jobs have the greatest difficulty adjusting. This type* *of retiree needs to detach from the job. They need to work on building alternative activities, and they need to be aware that making their retirement life really flourish will take them a little longer than others.*

Forced retirement. *Retirees who freely choose to retire have smoother adjustments. Retirees who felt pressured to leave the work environment typically have troublesome adjustments.*

Positive Factors. Conversely, a number of positive behavioral styles and personality factors can moderate the retirement process.

Coping styles. *Retirees who can effectively cope with stress have the best adjustment. From a mental perspective, those who assume full responsibility for their adjustment have more success with retirement. They do not blame others for their problems; they seek strategies for making their retirement process smooth and fully acceptable.*

Acceptance of challenge. *Retirees who accept the challenge of retirement instead of being overly fearful of change have the better adjustments. Retirement is a very challenging phase of life. It takes your full resources and full planning ability, but these efforts will pay off in a higher quality of life.*

Optimism and anticipation. *Retirees need optimism, even during rough times, and optimistic retirees adjust better than pessimists. People who view retirement with anticipation allow for a gradual adjustment over a period of time. Also, retirees whose jobs were stressful need to realize that they would have less stress once they are retired.*

■ The Optimal Retiree Profile ■

Some large-scale research studies have profiled retirees who made a quick, positive, three-month adjustment versus retirees who had a number of complications in the retirement process. Information from these studies can help you to better adjust to the retirement years.

Successful Retirees

Retirees who had optimal adjustment tended to have three things going for them. One, they had well-developed retirement plans; they did not shoot from the hip. Day in and day out they knew what they wanted to do; they had written it down, and they carried out these activities. Next, they maintained very positive attitudes toward retirement; full of optimism, they embraced the challenges ahead. Finally, retirees with a good program had an accurate idea of what retirement would be like; they were completely aware of all issues surrounding this new phase of life.

What were the scientific results of this study? Of retirees in this "successful adjustment" group, 71 percent grew accustomed to not working in three months' time, and they became used to their new lifestyle; 80 percent reported they were able to keep busy with meaningful activities; and 91 percent were fully satisfied with their retirement!

Unsuccessful Retirees

Researchers have also profiled "unsuccessful" retirees, those who had excessive difficulty with the retirement process. These people had a poor retirement program. Because they did not develop comprehensive retirement plans that they were committed to carrying out, they really did not know what they were going to do from one day to the next. After some initial vacations during the early days of retirement, their day-to-day routine became unplanned and unstructured. Next, they maintained an unfavorable attitude toward retirement, never fully accepting, mentally or emotionally, the challenge of this phase of life. Finally, the distressed retirees had an unclear, unrealistic perspective of retirement and what it would be like. They did not read books on retirement. They did not talk with retirees. They did not bother to pursue a good understanding of the retirement process.

And what did the result show? Of retirees with poorly developed programs, only 32 percent became adjusted in three months; fewer than 40 percent were able to keep busy with their day-to-day life activities; and only 54 percent were even "somewhat" satisfied with retirement. Obviously, these results are not as positive as the results of the retirees with a good program.

A statement by one respondent in the poor retirement program group really points out what happens when you do not build a strong retirement program. This is what he said:

Once you retire, you simply must find some kind of rewarding activity or you are sunk. There is a definite retirement vacuum, a state of dull, witless, and pointless idleness. I can speak for no one but myself, but I wish to God I was back on the job.

■
The Ultimate Recommendation
■

Many valuable employees, who could have provided years of useful work to society, have become physically ill and even prematurely incapacitated by having inadequate retirement plans and programs. This "psychosomatic illness," according to Dr. Hans Selye, the father of stress research, is so common that it has been given the name retirement disease.

This leads us into another retirement strategy: the best way to retire is to continue working! Identify a "work environment"—a community activity, a small company, some family project—that allows you to use some of the skills you routinely used before retirement. Identify suitable replacement activities where you do not have to learn a lot of new skills but, instead, can apply the wealth of skills you already know in a new, novel situation. If you are not sure what your skills are, a retirement counselor can help point them out.

Identify the work skills and activities that were most important and rewarding on your job. If you like to manage and delegate, then find an alternative work environment where you can manage and delegate. If you had a desire to learn a new facet of work, such as the use of computers, you now can seek training or schooling in this area. Be sure to select a replacement environment that fits your personality and needs. If you are a hard-driving executive, then you might not fit in with a social organization that does not value those skills. Instead, volunteer or begin a part-time job in some area where those skills can be utilized.

Begin to work in your replacement work environment, even if you set up an office in your own home where you can keep regular hours as you begin to work on some meaningful activity. Remember to give yourself time to find the most suitable "substitute work" environment.

Do not be afraid to change environments if you make a mistake, especially if you volunteer or choose a paid activity in an environment that you do not really like. Clearly, retirement has a definite psychological adjustment component. After all, your job occupied most of your waking hours for many years. It also satisfied many of your human needs.

■

Moving Ahead

■

Retirement is what you make of it. To summarize everything we've discussed above, you need to

- *Become educated about retirement (in addition to other resources, Appendix C provides a list of useful Web sites for retirees)*

- *Plan!*

- *Undertake meaningful activities*

- *Perceive adjustment to retirement as a challenge*

- *Most important, remain fully committed!*

- *Any adjustment to major life changes demands considerable personal effort. I invite you to accept this challenge.*

Appendix A

RETIREMENT STRESS INVENTORY (RSI)

This informal inventory rates *stressful changes* that have occurred in your life *within the last 12 months.* Nearly all of the events are either directly or indirectly related to the retirement process.

STEP 1

Circle a zero if the event did not occur. If a *change* did occur, indicate whether it was *tolerable* or *intolerable* by circling, respectively, the number 1 or 2 next to the question. Remember that even tolerable changes can trigger a stress response.

0 = Event did not occur

1 = Event occurred and was tolerable

2 = Event occurred and was intolerable

Which changes did you experience in the last 12 months?

---

1. Pressured by others to retire

    0   1   2

---

2. Offered incentives by company to retire

       0   1   2

3. Engaged in retirement planning

       0   1   2

4. Retired from job

       0   1   2

5. Spouse began or stopped work

       0   1   2

6. Financial status is a lot worse off

       0   1   2

7. Intend to take on a part-time or volunteer job

       0   1   2

8. Encountered legal problems (e.g., lawsuits)

      0   1   2

9. Increase in number of family arguments

      0   1   2

10. One or more children left home

      0   1   2

11. Increase in eating, smoking, or drinking habits

      0   1   2

12. Onset of serious illness or injury

      0   1   2

13. Divorce or separation

      0   1   2

14. Marriage or remarriage

          0   1   2

15. Change of residence

          0   1   2

16. Death of spouse

          0   1   2

17. Death of close family member

          0   1   2

18. Death of close friend

          0   1   2

19. Serious illness or injury of close family member

          0   1   2

20. Serious illness or injury of close friend

0   1   2

1	2

STEP 2. Sum the circled answers: *(column subtotals)*

STEP 3. Add up your total score *(it should range from 0 to 40)*

Inventory Interpretation

Score Range and Explanation*

31- 40

This is an extremely high level of retirement stress. You might be at high risk to experience physical and emotional distress. Medical and/or psychological counseling is usually recommended for scores this high.

21 - 30

You are experiencing an above-average level of distress. This level of retirement stress could be causing some emotional, social, and/or physical problems in your life. Clinical counseling appears relevant for scores in this range.

11 - 20

You are experiencing a number of challenging changes in your life that require strong coping skills. Although you might perceive many of these challenges as being tolerable, don't minimize the amount of stress that even desirable life changes can create. Counseling might be needed!

0 - 10

You are experiencing lower levels of retirement stress. However, it is still important to be able to cope with all forms and levels of stress, no matter how big or small.

Note: These are informal RSI interpretation guidelines. They should not be taken as definitive recommendations for medical or psychological counseling. Also, some of the RSI questions tend to be written for retirees with families and/or "significant others." Therefore RSI scores might be less meaningful for respondents who do not have any accessible family members or friends.

Appendix B

Progressive Relaxation Training:
A Stress Management Script for Retirees

The following script has been prepared to provide all interested *retirees* with sufficient information about progressive relaxation training so that they can learn this technique and employ it when experiencing unwanted tension. The following script is also relevant for other "high-risk" employees (e.g., frustrated managers, employees facing disruptive change, etc.). Progressive relaxation training is only one type of intervention that is included as an example.

Progressive relaxation is a skill that most retirees can benefit from learning. Also, most people in the preretirement stages experience some unwanted tension at various times in their lives. A large number of both retirees and preretirees likely can learn to cope more effectively with everyday pressures and tension by learning and practicing progressive relaxation.

Progressive relaxation training involves two basic components: (1) systematic tensing and releasing of various muscle groups throughout the body, and (2) learning to discriminate between the resulting sensations of tension and relaxation. **Learning progressive relaxation, therefore, is an active process that requires consistent, diligent practice. Acquisition of this skill is very much like learning to ride a bicycle, to swim, or to ski. That is, in order to get better, a person must practice!**

A Few Cautions

Progressive relaxation should not be viewed as a panacea or substitute for medical and/or psychological treatment. Before undertaking a relaxation regimen, retirees with tension-related disorders such as insomnia, tension head-aches, or backaches should consult with a physician or clinical psychologist about their concerns.

Also, relaxation training is not equivalent to participation in supportive counseling. Employees cannot expect progressive relaxation to alleviate psychological symptoms such as depression and anxiety, or their feelings of anger, lack of assertiveness, or discomfort around others. Moreover, retirees experiencing a significant level of emotional distress are encouraged to seek help from a medical or mental health professional rather than using relaxation training as a substitute for such help. However, relaxation training sometimes is used in conjunction with other procedures in counseling.

Goal of Progressive Relaxation

The goal of progressive relaxation is to help individuals reduce muscle tension in the body at any time they desire to do so. The systematic tensing and releasing of muscle groups facilitates this process because a large and noticeable reduction in tension occurs each time a *tension-release* cycle is completed. Individuals learn to discriminate between tension and relaxation and become more aware of their areas of tenseness. Over a period of time, individuals can learn to relax quickly and effectively without tensing and relaxing all muscle groups.

An enjoyable level of relaxation can be achieved with a few practice sessions. Daily practice over a four-week period is usually necessary to obtain longer-term benefits. However, a permanent habit of taking time out of every day for a relaxation session is an optimum goal.

During the first two weeks you practice progressive relaxation, it is recommended that you complete the tension-relaxation exercises in their entirety. After this two-week period, you may find that you are able to achieve a deep level of relaxation in some muscle groups without the tension-release cycle. Instead, you may be able to relax a particular muscle group simply by focusing upon releasing the muscle. Over time, a deep level of relaxation can be achieved with a minimum number of tension-release sequences. People may also find that the use of pleasant imagery facilitates their enjoyment of relaxation. Following mastery of the basic procedure, individual modifications of the procedure, to meet personal preferences, are encouraged.

In addition to daily practice, the following have been found helpful for those learning progressive relaxation:

- *Allow at least 30 minutes for your daily relaxation sessions.*

- *Try to arrange the relaxation session so that you are not interrupted during your half-hour of relaxation.*

- *Remove any restrictive clothing (tight belts, glasses, shoes, and wrist watches) before beginning a session.*

Assume a comfortable position in a reclining chair or lying on your back on a bed or soft rug. For most people, a comfortable position involves having (a) legs slightly apart; (b) arms away from the body, slightly bent at the elbows; (c) hands open, fingers slightly spread apart; (d) jaw slack, lips parted slightly; and (e) eyes closed.

Do not try to relax any muscle groups if you do not think you are physically capable of doing so. Simply listen to your tape and *imagine* yourself relaxing them. The following script covers the basic principles of progressive relaxation.

Relaxation Script

This script should be read into a personal recorder for playback. (You may need to record this script onto a longer-playing audiotape.) The reader should use a clear, soothing voice. The reader should take a slight pause whenever he or she encounters an ellipsis. You might select a friend or family member to record this script, or the reader might be you. Once completed, this audiotape should be played every time you engage in this form of relaxation. Now, *begin recording*.

Relaxation of Arms

Settle back and get as comfortable as you can. Let yourself relax to the best of your ability. Now, as you relax like that, clench your right fist. Just clench your fist tighter and tighter, and study the tension as you do so. Keep it clenched and feel the tension in your right fist, hand, forearm... Now, relax. Let the fingers of your right hand become loose, and observe the contrast in your feelings... Now, let yourself go and try to become more relaxed all over... Once again, clench your right fist really tight... Hold it, and notice the tension again... Now let go, relax. Let your fingers straighten out, and you should notice the difference once more... Now repeat the process with your left fist. Clench your left fist while the rest of your body relaxes, clench that fist tighter and feel the tension... And now, relax. Again enjoy the contrast... Repeat that once more. Clench the left fist, tight and tense... Now do the opposite of tension. Relax and feel the difference. Continue relaxing like that for awhile... Clench both fists tighter and tighter, both fists tense, forearms tense, study the sensations... and then relax. Straighten out your fingers and feel that relaxation.

Continue relaxing your hands and forearms more and more... Now bend your elbows and tense your biceps. Tense them harder and study the tension feelings... All right, straighten out your arms. Let them relax and feel the difference again. Let the relaxation develop... Once more, tense your biceps; then relax to the best of your ability... Each time, pay close attention to your feelings when you tense up and when you relax... Now straighten your arms; straighten them so that you feel most tension in the triceps muscles along the back of your arms. Stretch your arms and feel that tension... And now, relax. Let your arms fall back into a comfortable position. Let the relaxation proceed on its own. The arms once more should feel comfortably heavy as you allow them to relax... Straighten the arms once more so that you feel the tension in the triceps muscles; straighten them. Feel that tension... and relax.

Now let's concentrate on pure relaxation in the arms without tension. Get the arms comfortable and let them relax further and further. Continue relaxing your arms even further. Even when your arms seem fully relaxed, try to go that extra bit further; try to achieve deeper and deeper levels of relaxation.

Relaxation of Facial Area with Neck, Shoulders, and Upper Back

Relax your entire body to the best of your ability. Feel that comfortable heaviness. Let all your muscles go loose and heavy. Just settle back quietly and comfortably. Wrinkle up your forehead now; wrinkle it tighter... And now, stop wrinkling your forehead; relax and smooth it out. Picture the entire forehead and scalp becoming smoother as the relaxation increases... Now frown and crease your eyebrows and study the tension... Let go of the tension again. Smooth out the forehead once more... Now, close your eyes tighter and tighter. Feel the tension... and then relax your eyes. Keep your eyes closed, gently, comfortably, and notice the relaxation... Now clench your jaws; bite your teeth together. Study the tension throughout the jaws... Now, relax your jaws. Let your lips part slightly. Appreciate the relaxation... Now press your tongue hard against the roof of your mouth. Look for the tension... All right, let your tongue return to a comfortable and relaxed position... Now purse your lips; press your lips tighter and tighter... Relax the lips. Note the contrast between tension and relaxation.

Feel the relaxation all over your face, all over your forehead and scalp, eyes, jaws, lips, tongue and your neck muscles. Press your head back as far as it can go and feel the tension in the neck. Roll it to the right and feel the tension shift. Now roll it to the left. Straighten your head and bring it forward. Press your chin against your chest. Let your head return to a comfortable position, and study the relaxation. Let the relaxation develop... and just relax.

Now shrug your shoulders. Hold the tension... Drop your shoulders and feel the relaxation... Shrug your shoulders again. Feel the tension in your shoulders and in your upper back... Drop your shoulders once more and relax. Let the relaxation spread deep into the shoulders, right into your back muscles. Relax your neck and throat, your jaws, and other facial areas as the pure relaxation takes over and grows deeper... deeper... ever deeper.

Relaxation of Chest, Stomach, and Lower Back

Relax your entire body to the best of your ability. Feel that comfortable heaviness that accompanies relaxation. Breathe easily and freely in and out. Notice how the relaxation increases as you exhale... As you breathe out just feel that relaxation... Now breathe in and fill your lungs; inhale deeply and hold your breath. Study the tension... Now exhale. Let the walls of your chest grow loose and push the air out automatically. Continue relaxing and breathe freely and gently. Feel the relaxation and enjoy it... With the rest of your body as relaxed as possible, fill your lungs again. Breathe in deeply and hold it again... That's fine, breathe out and appreciate the relief. Just breathe normally. Continue relaxing your chest and let the relaxation spread to your back, shoulders, neck, and arms... Now merely let go. Enjoy the relaxation.

Now let's pay attention to your stomach area. Tighten your stomach muscles; make your abdomen hard. Notice the tension... and then relax. Let the muscles loosen and notice the contrast... Once more, press and tighten your stomach muscles. Hold the tension and study it... and relax. Notice the general well being that comes with relaxing your stomach... Now draw your stomach in, pull the muscles right in and feel the tension this way... Now relax again. Let your stomach out. Continue breathing normally and easily and feel this gentle massaging action all over your chest and stomach... Now pull your stomach in again and hold the tension... Now push out and relax... Once more, pull in and feel the tension... Now relax your stomach fully. Let the tension dissolve, as the relaxation grows deeper.

Each time you breathe out, notice the rhythmic relaxation both in your lungs and in your stomach. Notice how your chest and your stomach relax more and more... Try and let go of all contractions anywhere in your body.

Now direct your attention to your lower back. Gently arch your back upward. Make your lower back quite hollow, and feel the tension along your spine... And settle down comfortably again, relaxing the lower back... Just gently arch your back again and feel the tensions as you do so. Try to keep the rest of the body as relaxed as possible. Try to localize the tension throughout your lower back area... Relax once more, relaxing further and further. Relax your lower back, relax your upper back, and spread the relaxation to your stomach, chest, shoulders, arms, and facial area. Relax further and further and further and ever deeper.

Relaxation of Hips and Thighs

Let go of all tensions and relax... Now flex your buttocks and thighs. Flex your thighs by pressing down your heels as hard as you can... Relax and note the difference. Straighten your knees and flex your thigh muscles again. Hold the tension... Now, relax your hips and thighs. Allow the relaxation to proceed on its own. Press your feet and toes downward, away from your face, so that your calf muscles become tense. Study that tension... Relax your feet and calves... This time, bend your feet toward your face so that you can feel the tension along your shins. Bring your toes right up... Relax again... Now, let yourself relax further all over. Relax your feet, ankles, calves and shins, knees, thighs, buttocks, and hips. Feel the heaviness of your lower body as you relax still further... Now spread the relaxation to your stomach, waist, and lower back. Let go more and more deeply... Make sure that no tension has crept into your throat. Relax your neck and your jaw and all of your facial muscles. Keep relaxing your whole body like that for a while. Let yourself relax.

Complete Body Relaxation

Now you can become twice as relaxed as you are, merely by taking a really deep breath and slowly exhaling. With your eyes closed so that you become less aware of objects and movements around you, breathe in deeply and feel yourself becoming heavier. Take in a long, deep breath and let it out very slowly... Feel how heavy and relaxed you have become.

In a state of perfect relaxation, you should feel unwilling to move a single muscle in your body. Think about the effort that would be required to raise your right arm. As you think about raising your right arm, see if you can notice any tensions that might have crept into your shoulder and your arm... Now you can decide not to lift the arm but to continue relaxing. Observe the relief and the disappearance of the tension.

While you are relaxed like that, imagine a pleasant scene far away from hassles and daily pressures... For some people this might be a beautiful green meadow, soft and lush with abundant wild flowers... For another person, it may be the seashore at midday—the sun brilliant, pouring its warmth down on you; the waves lapping in and out, lulling you to sleep... Someone else might envision fishing on a quiet, dark lake in early morning—watching the sun rise, hearing the sounds of wildlife and of other people waking, appreciating the glow of a campfire burning on the shore... Choose a pleasant scene for yourself and appreciate this scene with all of your senses. Note the sights, sounds, smells, tastes, and textures of the scene. Enjoy this scene for the next minute or so.

Just carry on relaxing like that. When you wish to get up, count backward from four to one. You should then feel fine and refreshed, wide-awake and calm.

Appendix C

◼
Web Sites for Retirees
◼

General Sites

www.aarp.org

The *American Association for Retired Persons (AARP)* is the nation's leading organization for people age 50 and older. AARP serves their needs and interests through information, education, advocacy, and a sense of community.

www.aoa.dhhs.gov/elderpage.html#ap

Provides consumer information on a number of health issues of special concern to seniors, including health management, hearing services, and life extension. This site was put together by the *National Institutes of Health's National Institute on Aging*.

www.aoa.dhhs.gov/elderpage.html#ea

Supplies useful information on retirement-related topics such as fitness, volunteer opportunities, caregiving, depression, home adaptation, retirement living, mobility, vaccinations, and late-onset diabetes. This site is part of the *U.S. Administration on Aging's* home page.

www.epn.org/families.html

The *Families USA* section provides links to press releases and reports on Medicare, Medicaid and healthcare. This site also discusses the impact of proposed legislation on seniors. This site serves as a clearinghouse of medical information for seniors, too.

www.onlinenews.net/retirement.html

Provides comprehensive classifieds for retirees on retirement planning and communities.

Financial Sites

www.401kforum.com

The 401k Forum provides solutions to 401K planning.

www.fidelity.com

Fidelity Investments assists retirees with portfolio planning.

www.financialengines.com

Financial Engines provides general investment advice to retirees.

www.kiplinger.com

Covers financial issues related to retirement, and provides a videotape and newsletter on the topic.

www.quicken.com

Intuit provides general advice on financial planning and tax preparation for retirees.

www.vanguard.com

The Vanguard Group offers an online financial planning system for retirees.

References

Beck, S.H. (1982) Adjustment to and satisfaction with retirement. *Journal of Gerontology*, 37, 616-624.

Beehr, T.A. (1986) The process of retirement: A review and recommendations for future investigation. *Personnel Psychology*, 39(1), 31-55.

Dawis, R.V. and Lofquist, L.H. (1984) *A psychological theory of work adjustment: individual differences model and its applications.* Minneapolis: University of Minnesota Press.

Floyd, F.J., Doll, S.N., Winemiller, D., Lemsky, C., Burgy, T.M., Werle, M., and Heilman, N. (1992) Assessing retirement satisfaction and perceptions of retirement experiences. *Psychology and Aging*, 7, 609-621.

Fouquereau, E., Fernandez, A., and Mulet, E. (1999) The Retirement Satisfaction Inventory: Factor structure in a French sample. *European Journal of Psychological Assessment*, 15(1), 49-56.

Johnson, R.P. and Riker, H.C. (1981) Retirement maturity: A valuable concept for preretirement counselors. *Personnel and Guidance Journal*, January Issue, 291-295.

Jones, J.W. (1987) *High-level positive retirement: An education program for pre-retirement planning.* Arlington Heights, IL: BPRI Press. (WWW.BPRI.COM)

Kim, S. and Feldman, D.C. (1998) Healthy, Wealthy, or Wise: Predicting actual acceptance of early retirement incentives at three points in time. *Personnel Psychology,* 51(3), 623-642.

Maddi, S. and Kobasa, S. (1984) *The hardy executive: Health under stress.* Homewood, IL: Dow-Jones Irwin.

Menduno, M. (1999) Retirement plans go online. *The Industry Standard,* Aug 2-9, 51-58.

Mutran, E.J., Reitzes, D.C. and Fernandez, M.E. (1997) Factors that influence attitudes toward retirement. *Research on Aging,* 19(3), p. 251(23).

Selye, H. (1974) *Stress without distress.* Philadelphia: Lippincott.

Taylor Carter, M.A. and Cook, K. (1995) Adaptation to retirement: Role changes and psychological resources. *The Career Development Quarterly,* 44, 67-82.

Von Haller Gilmer, B. (1981) *Planning for retirement: A guide for managers.* Blacksburg, VA: Virginia Polytechnic Institute, Technical Report, pp. 1-25.

■
About the Author
■
■

The Everyday Psychologist who anonymously authored this book is a state licensed, Ph.D.-level professional. This author is an applied psychologist with training and certifications in the fields of clinical counseling, medical psychotherapy, and industrial psychology. This author has served as both an individual and a group psychotherapist, specializing in addiction therapy and the treatment of stress disorders. This psychologist first became exposed to the field of retirement psychology when he/she presented preretirement psychoeducational programs to executives and their families. This author observed firsthand how retirees and their families could achieve a high-level positive retirement by learning how to cope with retirement stress.

Another popular book in *The Everyday Psychology Series* is:

- **Spiritual Health Psychology:** *Profiling your Spiritual Self for Improved Health and Life Satisfaction (ISBN: 0-9668417-3-5)*